Bricks & Barbwire

R. J. Grigaitis, S.F.O.

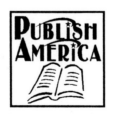

PublishAmerica
Baltimore

First printing

ISBN: 1-4137-5107-5
PUBLISHED BY PUBLISHAMERICA, LLLP
www.publishamerica.com
Baltimore

Printed in the United States of America

Contents

Sgt. Pepper's Lonely Hearts Club Band

Well, I've finally started it. I've been thinking and talking about this book for three years now, and I'm finally beginning to write it. Today is a very appropriate day to begin a work such as this. This is the tenth World Day of the Sick to be celebrated on the feast of Our Lady of Lourdes. It is appropriate because I am writing about sickness, specifically mental illness. More specifically, my mental illness: schizoaffective disorder.

I have waited this long before beginning to working on this book because I've been working on some other books that I wanted to finish before beginning this one (these other books have nothing to do with mental illness, but deal primarily with theology). Unfortunately, I have not had the cognitive faculties to work on these other books for over a year and a half now, so I've given up on these other books for the time being. I'm not going to worry too much about being overly cohesive in this book for two reasons: first, as I already said, my cognitive faculties are not fully functioning right now; and second, a lack of cohesiveness will reflect the way my mental illness affects my thinking sometimes.

A number of people have encouraged me in undertaking this task, especially my mental health nurse, and a good friend of mine that also works in the mental health field. I have been told that there are very few books written about mental illness by people that actually have a mental illness. This is one of reasons I am writing this book.

There are many other reasons as well. I want to help other people, and I want to help myself. Writing is a process that not only allows you to communicate to others, but also allow you to better understand what you are writing about. I have come to way better understanding of theology by writing about it. Way more than if I just read about it. By writing about my mental illness I hope to understand it better; define what it is and how it affects me; and learn to live with it better.

I also want others to better understand mental illness. I want to help those working in the mental health field to better understand what it's like to have a mental illness. The more they understand mental illness the better they can help us who have one.

As well, in giving people close to me a better understanding of how my mental illness has affected me, I hope they will be more sympathetic and tolerant of the strange things I have done. I have done many, many strange things, some of which I will describe in this book. Repeatedly, people will ask me about different things and I simply say, "I don't know," or try to change the topic. The reason I do this is because I am embarrassed to talk about some of the stuff I've done. If I did talk about it, I would have to take the time to explain my illness and how it affected me in these matters. Once this book is complete, instead of saying, "I don't know," or trying to change the topic, I can simply say, "Read my book."

The most important reason for writing this book is to let others like me know that they are not alone. From reading about, and watching videos on, mental illness the most helpful information to me are the insights where I say to myself, "This happens to me! I'm not alone!" I hope others will have experiences like this when they read this book, and know that they're not alone.

> Living now with feelings,
> Gives my life some meaning,
> Leaves in me a hope of things to come,
> Now I see I'm not the only one.

Occasionally throughout this book I will insert some song lyrics. Music is a very important way that I express myself, and I will quote some of the songs I have written.

I would like to keep this book really generic, but that would be impossible. First of all, each person is unique and it would be unrealistic to think I could give a generic description of my mental illness. Plus, religion has played a very big part in my acceptance of my suffering, and a description of my mental illness would be very incomplete without describing a little of my faith journey. Nonetheless, I will try to limit my description of my faith journey to details pertinent to my mental illness.

I will try to be historically accurate, but I know from experience that history is subject to error. The experience I'm talking about is listening to others describe shared experiences inaccurately. I'm sure my version of history is correct, but I'm humble enough to recognise that I'm just as susceptible to historical error as everyone else (actually, I really do think my version of history is the right one).

Additionally, as the word *mental* in the term *mental illness* implies, this illness affects the mind. One of the affects it has had on my mind is that large portions of my memory are blank just before, during, and shortly after my hospitalisations. I'm sure the ECTs (electroconvulsive therapy) didn't help this much either. I do remember some things from this time period, and others have filled me in a bit, so I'll try to be as historically accurate as I can be concerning these blank and fuzzy areas in my memory.

There are some historical facts, however, that I do not wish to bring up. This may be because they are too sensitive to me, but mostly because I don't want to hurt others. Some of what I write may be upsetting to some, but I'll try to keep this to a minimum. In these cases I may just give a general description with a few choice details left out.

Please don't interpret what I write as blaming others for my problems. Everyone in my life has done the best they could to help me. It's true that everyone in my life failed to help me until my first hospitalisation, but I know that they failed me due to their ignorance.

It is important to take into consideration the date and location of my early history. I was born on the second anniversary of the British release of the Beatles album *Sgt. Pepper's Lonely Hearts Club Band*, in a small town on the Canadian prairies. I began grade school in the mid '70s and finished high school at the end of the '80s. Since this time, public awareness of mental illness has improved a great deal, and I hope that children such as myself do not have to wait thirty years before receiving the help they need.

I was twenty-nine and a half years old before I received the help I needed. My wife and my mother took me to the hospital, where I was admitted and taken to the lock down ward. At first I was diagnosed with bipolar affective disorder, but this diagnosis was later changed to schizoaffective disorder.

Schizoaffective disorder is basically schizophrenia and clinical depression or bipolar disorder together (in my case it's clinical depression). Clinical depression can produce profound feelings of sadness, loneliness, hopelessness, and worthlessness. It can also be responsible for fatigue and loss of energy (it was nice to find out that I was clinically depressed and not lazy). Between 10% to 15% of people with clinical depression commit suicide.

Schizophrenia produces unusual or bizarre thinking and behaviour. Including in this thinking and behaviour are paranoia, delusions, hallucinations, and withdrawal from reality and society. Roughly half the people with schizophrenia attempt to commit suicide, of which around a quarter will succeed.

Sex

As I said in the first chapter, so as not to hurt others, there are some historical facts that I do not wish to write about. My sexual past is one of these. Before and during my hospitalisations, I sought counselling to help me deal with my sexual past. I now feel at peace with my sexual past, and it no longer has a hold on me. I strongly urge all those who have influenced me sexually, and all those who I have influenced sexually, to seek professional help.

I say *influenced sexually* because I believe I have not been sexually abused, nor have I sexually abused anyone else. For sexual abuse to take place, either an adult would have to be involved, or someone would have to be forced to act against his or her own will. All of my sexual experiences have been with consenting parties, who were only a few years older or younger than myself.

These damaging sexual experiences began when I was around four or five years old, and compounded the symptoms of my mental illness. The bizarre thinking and behaviour caused by my mental illness often centred on my sexuality. Although I am not going to write about it, the results of my sexual past coupled with my mental illness have tormented me more than anything else.

Again, I strongly urge all those who have influenced me sexually, and all those who I influenced, to seek professional help. I do not blame you for my problems. I know you were acting out of ignorance.

> Like a child, lonely and confused,
> Like a child, broken and abused,
> Like a child, like a child, like a child.

Living out my life, knowing it ain't right,
Not knowing what to do, when I think of you,
The pain starts coming through,
feeling…
Like a child, lonely and confused,
Like a child, broken and abused,
Like a child, like a child, like a child.
Loss of innocence, lack of confidence,
It cuts me to the heart, not knowing who's the start,
It pierces like a dart,
to feel…
Like a child, lonely and confused,
Like a child, broken and abused,
Like a child, like a child, like a child.
You took my trust away, what was I to say,
You were the world to me, you brought me to my knee,
How was I to see,
you were…
Like a child, lonely and confused,
Like a child, broken and abused,
Like a child, like a child, like a child.

There is one point though that I should mention to set the record straight. I am very much a heterosexual, and I have not had any homosexual experiences. The reason my sexual orientation may be questioned is because in high school it became popular among a certain group of friends to jokingly act gay. I found out a few years later that not everyone knew this was only a joke. As well, I now question whether or not some of these guys were joking.

As well, I should point out that despite all my damaging sexual experiences, I lost my virginity to my wife, who is the only person I have ever had sexual intercourse with.

Since my wife left me, I've had to come to terms with being celibate. At first it was very hard for me to accept, but now I embrace the celibate life. I feel more fulfilled in celibacy than when I was sexually active. I can remarry because I am divorced and my marriage has been annulled, but I won't because I feel called to remain celibate. I now understand and accept the words of Christ in Matthew 19:12: "Some are born incapable of marriage. Others have been made that way by men. But there are others who have given up the possibility of marriage for the sake of the kingdom of Heaven. He who can accept this, let him accept it." [1]

I have accepted it.

[1] Christian Community Bible, 2nd Edition. Philippines: Claretian Publications, St. Paul Publications, & Divine Word Publications, 1988

Drugs

It is very common for people with a mental illness to *self-medicate*. That is, to seek relief from the symptoms of their mental illness with alcohol or street drugs. Most of the time they are not conscious that they are doing this. I can definitely see this in looking back on my life, although I was never conscious that I was trying to combat the symptoms of my mental illness.

My first encounter with drugs was when I was in the early grades of elementary school. A second cousin of mine stopped by the house when my parents were not home. He offered to take me for a ride on his motorcycle, which I accepted. The motorcycle ride was uneventful, with the exception of the thrill of riding on a motorcycle, but later that day, my mom explained to me that it was dangerous to go anywhere with him because he uses drugs.

I don't remember my mom's explanation of what drugs were, but it did make an impression on me. I realised drugs were bad; however, a curiosity about them arose in me. My mom has told me that I made a comment about putting everyone that uses drug someplace away from everyone else so they don't hurt anyone. I guess my idea would be along the lines of a cross between a hippie commune and a penal colony.

As time went on, my curiosity about drugs grew. On the farm where I lived, there was what used to be the old highway that led to what we called *the Picnic Spot* (the high school kids referred to it as *Where The F**k Are We*). We would often go to this spot to collect beer bottles to take to the bottle depot. Occasionally we would find drug paraphernalia here, such as a hash pipe that my dad found that was made of a toilet paper roll and tinfoil. I remember pretending with my sister that I was a drug users, making a hash pipe like the one my dad found. Once we even found a small garden of marijuana. If I had found this garden a couple of years later, I would have used it myself. As it was, my dad phoned the police, and they came and collected the produce.

One thing that really fuelled my curiosity about drugs was a booklet that my mom bought. The idea behind the booklet was to educate kids about drugs to prevent them from trying them. The book was very detailed, filled with pictures of drugs and drug paraphernalia. This book had the opposite effect on me than what was intended.

During the summer prior to grade eight, a pivotal event took place in my life: I discovered Rock 'n' Roll, specifically, the Beatles. While I will talk about this more in the next chapter, reading about the Beatles and their drug use only increased my curiosity in drugs.

I was still a little scared of drugs, so, in imitation of the Beatles, I decided to experiment with Transcendental Meditation, which was suppose to achieve the same results as drugs. I didn't really know what I was doing with Transcendental Meditation. There was no way I would fork out the cash necessary to learn how to do it properly, and there was no way my mother would allow me enroll in any Transcendental Meditation classes. I was not in the least bit interested in receiving a genuine Transcendental Meditation mantra since, from a Christian perspective, these mantras invoked demons. It wasn't long before I abandoned the idea of achieving a mystical state of mind with Transcendental Meditation, and I began to think more seriously about trying drugs.

Around this time, I got drunk for the first time. I don't really want to get into all the details of this event because I was only fifteen at the time, and I don't want to incriminate the person I was drinking with, especially since he was driving under the influence. I will say a couple of things though. First, I really liked being drunk. It felt very liberating. I think that it did alleviate some of the symptoms of my mental illness, even though I was not aware I had a mental illness.

This first time under the influence of alcohol also revealed the way alcohol affected me; or should I say, the lack of affect it had on me. As

I said, I liked drinking, so I pour myself a couple of drinks without my drinking partner knowing it. As well, he gave me his drink to finish before we drove to the bar to pick up a six pack. Despite the fact that he was more than twenty years my senior, and was almost twice my body weight, at the end of the evening he was drunker than I was.

Another thing began to influence me at this age: other kids in school began trying drugs. Not only were drugs a way to achieve a mystical state of mind, they were *cool*. At this time, being cool was one of the most important things for me to do, so actually doing drugs was not as important as having the reputation of doing drugs.

One day, someone at school was passing out candy cigarettes. I ate the candy, but saved the paper. I took the paper home and stuffed dried parsley in it, and smoked it the next day.

My next experiment was to take a small tray of dried parsley and soak it with gin. Over a few days I let the gin evaporate. I somehow thought that the gin would evaporate and leave alcohol in the parsley, which I then smoked.

I also tried smoking catnip, sniffing rubber cement, and sniffing gasoline.

When I finally decided to buy real drugs at the end of grade nine, I ended up at the police station with my parents. This experience scarred me enough that I decided to have nothing to do with drugs. Aside from getting drunk a few more times, I stayed away from drugs until my grade eleven year.

In grade eleven I began spending most of my Saturdays with an older group of friends, and most of these Saturdays involved getting high. It was primarily marijuana that we did: grass, hash, and hash oil; although we did do mushrooms a few times.

The summer after grade eleven I began toking-up quite regularly, pretty much every weekday at work, and sometimes on the weekend. After that summer I became very serious about my drumming (more on that in the next chapter), and I slowed down my cannabis intake quite a bit. It was only the occasional weekend that I would either get drunk or get high. As I said, alcohol didn't affect me too much, so I preferred getting high since it was a better value for my money.

After grade twelve, I returned to high school for one more semester. By this time, a couple of my friends had tried acid (lysergic acid diethylamide, better known as LSD), and I was thinking of trying it. Despite the pleadings of one of my best friends, I decided to give acid a try. This was the drug that I had been most curious about for the last five years. A friend of mine was going to score me some acid, and I was going to score him some hash. I got the hash, but he failed to get the acid. So I smoked the hash with someone else, and I never did try acid. Although I'm sure some sort of hallucinogenics were mixed in with some of the grass and hash that I've smoked.

Looking back, I'm sure that the hand of God was in this. Now that I know how ill my mind is, I'm sure acid would have sent me off the deep end and I may not have come back.

The last time I got stoned was Thursday, November 10, 1988, but this story actually starts two weeks before this. A friend and I went to a laser light show, and got really, really stoned on hash. This is one of the times that I believe that some sort of hallucinogenics were mixed with the stuff we smoked. During the show I had an extremely intense mystical experience in which God told me to stop using drugs, after which my deceased grandfather told me that he was very disappointed that I was using drugs, and that I should stop. The show itself was incredible, although I think I had my eyes closed throughout most of it.

The next weekend I got stoned on a whole handful of pills, mostly pain killers with codeine. This was not a fun night. It was the first and only time I had a bad high. Towards the end of the evening, I actually thought I was going to die. The thought of death really scared me because the way I was living was not a Christian life, and therefore, I was not dying a Christian death. The thought of going to Hell was much scarier than my earlier incident at the police station. I vowed to God that if I lived I would stop using drug.

I'm not sure whether my life was really in danger; however, despite this possible brush with death, I got stoned again the following weekend. This was a long weekend; November 11th is Remembrance Day in Canada, which means that that Friday was a holiday, which meant that that Thursday was a good night to have a party. There was one problem though: my drum lessons were on Thursday nights. In my rush to go out and buy some grass, I completely forgot about my drum lesson.

On my way to the party after buying the grass, I stopped at home. My sister informed me that everyone was wondering where I was because I was supposed to be at my drum lesson. I couldn't do anything about it now, so I went to the party and got really, really stoned again.

This was really strong grass. I'm sure that some sort of hallucinogenics were mixed in with this stuff as well. I had never been this stoned before. It was great! I could actually taste the colours in ginger ale. It was so strong that I was still stoned the next morning and into the rest of that day. As I was driving home, I began to have another profound mystical experience. It was so strong that I had to pull off to the side of the road. During this mystical experience, God again told me to stop using drugs.

After this weekend, I did a lot of serious thinking. Twice God told me to stop using drugs, I almost died, and I missed a drum lesson. At this time in my life, drumming was number one on my list of priorities. Were drugs replace drumming as number one? This may seem odd, but I stopped using drugs because they jeopardised my career as a musician. That is, illegal drugs, I still drank occasionally.

Once I was married and had kids, my drinking was restricted to two or three drinks on special occasions. This changed, however, once my illness began to over power me. During the summer before my hospitalisations, I had a very strong craving for alcohol. This craving was satisfied at a wedding where I had around a dozen or more drinks. This may seem like a lot, but with the way my body handles alcohol, I was only a little bit tipsy. My children were with me, and I didn't want to become truly drunk in their presence. This was a clear case of self-medicating.

Since my hospitalisations, every time the symptoms of the illness get unbearable, I crave drugs and alcohol. I haven't satisfied these cravings with drugs, although I would like to. A few times I have had a little to drink, just enough to take the edge off reality. I would like to drink more, but I try to control myself.

A lot of times I feel like an alcoholic. I need a drink. It takes all my strength to resist this temptation. I am by myself a lot, so I could buy myself a bottle, get drunk, and no one would know. I am scared to do this though. I know that if I do it once, nothing would stop me from doing it again, and again, and again…

I know of an older gentleman who is an alcoholic. He stays in his apartment all day long, and every week his son brings him a couple mickeys of vodka. At times I'm envious of this man. I would like to withdraw from society and get drunk all the time.

This is a hard cross to bear. I know that drugs and alcohol are not the answer to my problems, but it sure would be an easy way out.

And Rock 'n' Roll

Most young people, especially teenagers, like to define who they are by the music they listen to, and I'm no exception. Like most young children, aside from children's records, I listened to the music my parents listened to. My mom liked country, and my dad liked classical. When I was young, my favourite two records were *Keep On Truckin'* and *Eine Kleine Nachtmusik*. My mom has told me that when I got overly upset or frustrated, she would sit me down on the couch, put *Eine Kleine Nachtmusik* on the record player, and I would settle right down.

Once I started grade one, the musical tastes of other kids began to influence me. The big group at that time was Kiss. A few kids in my class had older brothers, and they would bring their Kiss records to school. More than anything, I wanted a Kiss record. It wasn't that I really liked Kiss, but that I wanted what all the other kids had. I had a G. I. Joe and Six Million-Dollar Man action figures, and now I needed a Kiss record. My mom really didn't like the album covers on any of the Kiss records, so she bought me a 45 that didn't have a picture on the cover. I listen to it a bit, but I still preferred *Keep On Truckin'* and *Eine Kleine Nachtmusik*.

In 1977, Elvis Presley died. Before this time, I had never heard of Elvis. When I asked who Elvis was, my mom took out a couple of old records she had of his. As soon as I heard him I was hooked. My mom didn't mind buying me Elvis records; he looked a lot more pleasant than Kiss did.

After I had begun to listen to Elvis, I began to cry when I went to bed. When my mom would come in to see what the problem was, I would say, "Why did Elvis have to die?" She would comfort me and try to stop me from crying. Now, as I look back, something was not right here. I was upset over the death of a person I didn't know, and didn't even know existed until after his death. I had a grandfather who died a couple of years earlier, but I didn't cry over him. What would give me a reason to cry over Elvis?

I believe that I was crying over Elvis' death to receive attention. I was not seeking attention because of a lack of attention; both of my parents gave me ample attention. I think the problem was that, due to my mental illness, I could not fully absorb the attention I was receiving.

This was not the only thing I was doing for attention. When I was seven or eight, I fell out of a tree and hurt my back. My back was hurt so bad that it was very painful to stand. My parents took me to a chiropractor who gave me instant relief. This was the beginning of my chronic back problem.

It seemed that pretty much every time I fell down my back would go out and I couldn't walk. My back truly was out of alignment, but I seriously question my not being able to walk except for the first time. Once I fell down while cross-country skiing with my dad to the Picnic Spot. I claimed that I couldn't ski anymore. After trying a few things to get me home, my dad left me there to go get a toboggan to take me home on. It began to get dark and after a while, and I didn't want to be by myself in the woods anymore. I got up and began to run (you see, I really could stand). I went around fifty or seventy feet before I heard my mom and dad coming. I fell to the ground and told them that I was trying to crawl home.

Once I got old enough that it was embarrassing to have my dad to carry me, my back would simply go out, but not so bad that I couldn't walk. I really did have a chronic back problem, but I used it to get attention.

There were a number of other things I would do to get attention, such as hyperventilating. It was not because I lacked attention, but that I couldn't absorb the attention I was receiving. I can see this over and over again right up to my first hospitalisation.

By the way, I don't have a chronic back problem anymore. It went away once I began to regularly work-out with weights. I firmly believe that the best thing you can do for a chronic back problem is heavy deadlifts. Deadlifts strengthen the muscles in your back, and teach you how to lift properly.

In addition to Elvis, in grades three and four, I began listening to Abba, just like all the other kids; but I liked to emphasise that I listen to classical music. This again was an attention getter, this time the attention of my peers.

Emphasising that I listen to classical music worked as an attention getter in elementary school, but not in junior high. From grade two until grade six, I went to school with basically the same group of kids. In grade seven I was thrown into a class of strangers. Only three kids from my grade six class were in my grade seven class, and these were kids that I didn't really hang around with.

To say that I didn't fit-in in grade seven would be an understatement. I really didn't fit-in in elementary school, but the kids were more or less tolerant of my non-conformance. The reason for my non-conformance was my mental illness. I didn't know how to really conform and fit in, but more on that later.

I had no friends in grade seven. I really mean absolutely NO friends! For the whole year! I was the one everyone picked on. It would have helped if I started to listen to Ozzy Osbourne and Def Leppard instead of Beethoven and Luciano Pavarotti, but I didn't realise that this would be a ticket to acceptance.

Music only personified the way I didn't fit into society. Even when I started listening to Ozzy Osbourne and Def Leppard, I really didn't fit in, although I was somewhat socially accepted.

As I said in the last chapter, during the summer prior to grade eight, a pivotal event took place in my life: I discovered Rock 'n' Roll (by my standards Elvis and Abba aren't really Rock 'n' Roll), specifically, the Beatles. This was just before I had my braces removed, and my mom was taking me to the city quite regularly for my orthodontist appointments (remember, I lived in a small town, the city was a half-hour drive north of us). While we were in the city I decide to start taking records out of the city's library. I was only interested in classical music, but one day I said to my self, "I've heard of the Beatles. I wonder what they sound like?"

The Beatles record I took out was *Rarities*. I listened to the record with my sister. The first few songs, such as "Love Me Do," "Misery," "And I Love Her," were pretty good I thought. Then came the song "I Am the Walrus." My sister said, "This is weird!" I agreed, and said, "Yeah! I like it!" After that I was hooked. I took out all the Beatles records that that library had, as well as a couple Rolling Stone records, a Led Zeppelin record, and a record by the Who (yes, I was pirating).

I did like the Beatles' early stuff, but I preferred their later stuff, especially the stuff that was influenced by their use of acid. My favourite album was *Revolver*, of which my favourite song was "Tomorrow Never Knows."

For a grade twelve English project, I was supposed to take a poem or song lyrics and create a collage around the words. I painted the paper with a bunch of psychedelic designs and colours around the lyrics to "Tomorrow Never Knows." In a dozen places in the collage, I hid the letters "LSD" somewhat subliminally. I received a very high mark on this project. My teacher thought it was very clever to have the letters "LSD" all over it, and ask the other students if they could find all twelve occurrences. I thought she was nuts! I'm sure she didn't know what LSD really was.

Some people may not agree with me, but I believe that this type of music does create a mild psychedelic high. At least it does if you "turn off your mind, relax, and float down stream," "lay down all thoughts surrender to the void," and "listen to the colour of your dreams." Again, this is another example of self-medicating, this time with music rather than with alcohol or drugs.

Now I could be wrong, and this may be a symptom of my illness. Normal people may not be affected by music the same way it affects me. I don't know. What do you think?

Grade eight was much better than grade seven. I still didn't have any real friends, but I was socially accepted. The combination of talking about the Beatles and drugs, generally acting weird, and a different group of kids took me out of the role as the class's emotional punching bag. In this group of kids, only two were from my grade seven class, and these two never picked on me in grade seven. As well, I knew six of the kids in my grade eight class from elementary school. In all, this was the beginning of me becoming popular.

I found that being popular meant putting on a façade. Weird was good. Being somewhat of a clown was also good. Of course putting on a façade stopped anyone from actually getting to know me.

Part of the façade was a nickname I created, *Wall-Russ*. I thought that "I Am The Walrus" was a very cool song, and so I wanted people to call me the *Walrus*. I modified the spelling to match the shorten version of my name, *Russ*.

At the end of grade eight, I made another discovery, Heavy Metal. At the end of the school year, my junior high school would take all the kids to a near by beach. A number of kids brought ghetto blasters, and the main album that was being played was *Bark at the Moon* by Ozzy Osbourne. I really like the ballad on that record, "So Tired." That day I also heard a cover of the Beatles song "Helter Skelter."

The next day I went to the local record store and asked for the Ozzy Osbourne album that had "Helter Skelter" on it. I was then informed that that it was Mötley Crüe that did the cover of "Helter Skelter." I then asked for the Ozzy Osbourne album that had "So Tired" on it. He was all out of *Bark at the Moon*, so he sold me *Diary Of A Madman*. Again I was hooked. Ozzy led to Van Halen, Judas Priest, Iron Maiden, and all of the other Heavy Metal bands.

My façade changed to that of a head banger and stoner. As I said in the last chapter, it wasn't important that I had not actually tried drugs as much as it was that I gave the impression that I did. Looking back, I can see that most of the kids saw right through this thin veneer and I was the butt of a lot of jokes.

When I actually did try buying real drugs, I ended up at the police station with my parents. My parents attributed this rebellion as a result of this Heavy Metal music I was listening to, so they took away all of my Heavy Metal tapes for a month or two. What was I left with? The Beatles! It's kind of funny: to punish me for trying drugs they took away one kind of music, but left me with the music that really sparked my interest in drugs in the first place.

By the time I started grade ten, I was tired of the stoner image, and I wanted to be myself. I pretty much disposed of my façade as much as anyone could with schizophrenia, and I actually made some friends. Most of these friends were musicians, and it was in the context of jammin' together that our relationship was based (I played drums).

Throughout high school my musical tastes broadened a great deal. I listened to different styles of rock, from U2 to Metallica; different styles of jazz, such as Dave Brubeck, Weather Report, and Duke Ellington; progresive rock, like Yes and Frank Zappa; blues and R & B; reggae; latin; country; as well as baroque and classical. This musical diversity allowed me to have friends in a number of different cliques.

Since at this time I was self-medicating with street drugs, I was also able to self-medicate with music better, and I really like to combine the affects of drugs with those of music. Once I had stopped doing drugs, I continued to get high on music. Getting high on only music was much more successful after my experimenting with street drugs than it was before.

One record that I really liked to get high on was *4AD* by Bauhaus. This record was meant to be played at 45 rpm, but I didn't know that, and I played it at 33 1/3 rpm, which made it sound even more psychotic. I especially like the song "Rosegarden Funeral Of Sores," which was very depressive and psychotic, particularly when played at the slower speed. Even after I found out that it was supposed to be played at 45, I continued to play it at 33 1/3.

After high school I was accepted into the music program at a college in the city. After a couple of months I was beginning to come to the realisation that I didn't want to have a career in music. I spent more time on the phone to my girlfriend than I did studying and practising drums.

My girlfriend and I were talking seriously about marriage, and I was thinking that music was not a good career for a family man. Then my girlfriend became pregnant, which was a good excuse to dropout of the music program so I could find a job. After half a year working at various jobs that didn't pay too much, I went back to school to get a diploma in computer engineering.

Shortly before my wedding, I became very serious about

Christianity, and I began to listen to Christian music. The first time I really listened to Christian rock was while I was backing my brother-in-law's car out of the garage. I had listen to Christian rock before, my mom had even bought me a couple of tapes, but I never really paid much attention to it. In my brother-in-law's tape deck was the first Allies album. It caught my attention right away because the guitar solo was in the same style as Randy Rhoads (the guitarist on Ozzy's first two solo albums).

Since it was the first time that I was really living my faith, I started buying all sorts of Christian music. I kind of went a bit over board, and I now regularly listen to less than half of the Christian rock albums I've bought, although I did listen to them a lot when I first bought them.

After a year or so of only listening to Christian rock, I began to question the morality of listening to secular music. I took pretty much all my old records, tapes, and related books and paraphernalia, packed them in a big box, and stored them at my mom's place on the farm. I did keep some baroque and classical albums, and one gospel album by Elvis. However, I even packed up my Luciano Pavarotti.

After leaving these records in storage for a year, I went and burnt them all. Now on the surface it may look like I burnt these records because they conflicted with my faith, but that is not entirely correct. Most of the lyrics on these albums didn't conflict with my faith, although a few unquestionably did. This was not the first time I burnt stuff like this. I felt that these records had some sort of control over me, and the only way I could escape from their control was to burn them.

As I said, this was not the first time I burnt stuff like this, nor was it the last. In the same manner I burnt all my books by J. R. R. Tolkien, my books and magazines on martial arts, my books and magazines on motorcycles, even some obsolete computer equipment I had in storage, as well as a few other things. In all these cases I felt that these objects had control over me.

Now I'm not talking about the normal control objects have over people, where they are seeking happiness through material goods, which Christians try to avoid. I'm talking about real control, like a bridled horse, or a dog on a leash. The control that these records had on me was even stronger than that of the other objects because I could get somewhat of a high on some of this music. I wanted freedom from these records, as well as the other objects, so I burnt them all.

I'm glad I burnt some of these records, as I would not want my kids listening to them, or even looking at the covers, but most of them were harmless, and I wish I still had them. I also wish I still had my books by J. R. R. Tolkien, my books and magazines on martial arts, and especially my books and magazines on motorcycles. The only consolation I have is that most of this music was on vinyl, and I don't even own a record player anymore. Although there were two LPs that would still be worth having: I had Mike Stern's autograph on the cover of one of his records; and I had a rare copy of *Introducing The Beatles* released by Vee-Jay Records that had not even been taken out of the package yet. This last one would have been worth a fare bit of money, but it's gone now. Since my hospitalisations I have repurchased on CD a few of these record that I burnt, but only ones that I would let my kids listen to.

Music doesn't seem to have the same effect on me as it did before. I now only listen to music for enjoyment, and to relax. I don't listen to it anymore to create a high. I've even taken some Beatles and Jimi Hendrix CDs out of the library, but they don't affect me the way they used to.

All You Need Is Love

In the last chapter I said that I couldn't fully absorb the attention I was receiving; the same could be said for love. My illness prevents me from fully experiencing love, as it does all feelings. However, with the help of medications, I have come closer to experiencing love, especially in between my first and second hospitalisations.

From a very early age, I can see that I've been on a quest for love, not realising that my illness prevented me from absorbing the love that surrounds me. I was not able to absorb my parent's love, so I sought love outside my immediate family. The type of relationship that I attempted to find love in was the man-woman relationship, which was not so much love, as it was infatuation.

I was four years old when I had my first girlfriend. We were in tiny tots together, and I would be content to sit on a chair and watch her paint. I would play with her, but I remember quite vividly sitting on a chair and watching her paint for quite a long period of time, while my mom and teacher thought it was cute. It may have seemed cute, but this was an indication that something was wrong with me.

From tiny tots up to grade twelve, I searched for love over and over again with different girls, until I found my wife, who seemed to break through my emotional brick wall a little bit, and allow me to almost feel loved.

I look at you every morning
When I rise. I close my eyes
And I pray that you're safe
Through the day. How I wish to stay,

And leave the worries of the world
alone. I want to stay at home.
To be with you. To be with you.
To be with you, My love.
To be with you. To be with you.
To be with you, My love.
But I must go into this world
To provide so we survive.
And live with each other,
To hold and share the load.
And in the evening when the day is through,
I can be where I want to be.
To be with you. To be with you.
To be with you, My love.
To be with you. To be with you.
To be with you, My love.
I can't wait for all these days
To be through. To be with you
With the Father and the Son
And the Holy Ghost. I want the most
Beautiful Woman
To be with me.
To be with me. To be with me.
To be with me, My love.
To be with you. To be with you.
To be with you, My love.

Around a year and a half after my second hospitalisation, my wife left me. It would be uncharitable for me to discuss this topic here, but it was due to my illness that she left. The stress of living with me caused her to become physically ill. When she left me, she took away one of the few sources of love that I have been able recognise and receive.

You have filled my life with love
 You're a gift to me from above
 Now that you're gone I can't go on
 I need to live within your love
 Loneliness is what I feel
 An emptiness that only you can fill
 All I want is to hold you once again
 Please accept my song of love
 All my life I've been searching
 Been searching for your love
 Now that I found you I need you
 I need to live within your love
 Loneliness is what I feel
 An emptiness that only you can fill
 All I want is to hold you once again
 Please accept my song of love
 The sight of you fills me with bliss
 Just like the day of our first kiss
 All I can say is "I love you!"
 I need you to live within my love
 Loneliness is what I feel
 An emptiness that only you can fill
 All I want is to hold you once again
 Please accept my song of love

For the longest time after she left, I was convinced that one day she would return. This is what I yearned for more than anything else, save my yearning for the will of God, which I was sure was that our marriage be reconciled and our family be made whole.

I wake up this morning
I wake up from dreaming of you
I reach out to hold you, darling
That's when the pain starts coming through
An empty pillow in my bed
Thoughts of you running through my head
Come and rest your pretty head
On the pillow in my bed
The morning seems so empty
To wake up all alone
My heart feels so heavy
As heavy as a stone
An empty pillow in my bed
Thoughts of you running through my head
Come and rest your pretty head
On the pillow in my bed
I lie here thinking of you
Of our first night together
How I held you as you slept, dear
That's the best night I remember
An empty pillow in my bed
Thoughts of you running through my head
Come and rest your pretty head
On the pillow in my bed

It's now been almost four years since she left me. We are divorced, and our marriage has been annulled. It has been very hard for me to accept this, but I have accepted it. Once the annulment was final, I quit wearing my wedding ring, and gave up all hope for reconciliation. There's no animosity between us, and I harbour no resentment towards her. We are still friends, and we both want nothing more than what's best for our children.

It is the relationship with my children that has allowed me to feel the most love. I am their daddy, and they want to spend time with me. Many times I have profound feelings of loneliness were I feel nobody wants my company, but this never happens with my children. They always want my company, and I can recognise this.

My inability to receive love also hampers my relationship with God. My relationship with God is more of an intellectual one rather than a loving one. But my relationship with my children has helped me to accept God's love for me.

The last chapter also describes my quest for love among my peers. My bad experience in grade seven exemplifies my inability to connect with others. I do associate with a number of people, but I can't seem to establish a strong connection with them. I know that many people would be interested to establish a strong relationship with me, but I am unable to recognise these relational opportunities, and I remain primarily friendless.

I do have one friend that I've kept from high school, but even in this relationship I find it hard to recognise the closeness of the relationship. Emotionally I find it hard to recognise the relationship, although I can intellectually recognise the relationship. The concrete proof of this relationship is that I am the godfather of this friend's child, and I was actually asked to be the godfather after my hospitalisations and after my wife left me. If it were not for this concrete proof, I would not be able to accept the love from this friend.

With the help of medications, I have come closer to experiencing love, and I hope to continue to experience love more fully.

Living now with feelings,
Gives my life some meaning,
Leaves in me a hope of things to come,
Now I see I'm not the only one.
Live my life in pain, I'll never want again.
Not knowing how to love, or receiving of.
I must give it a chance, here I'll make my stance,

I'm receiving love.
Living now with all of me,
The road ahead a mystery,
Now I want to live my life in full,
Sick of putting up with all the bull.
Live my life in pain, I'll never want again.
Not knowing how to love, or receiving of.
I must give it a chance, here I'll make my stance,
I'm receiving love.

Suicide Solution

At the end of the first chapter I stated that roughly half the people with schizophrenia attempt to commit suicide, of which around a quarter will succeed. I have never attempted suicide, although I have been very, very close to doing so. I know, without a shadow of a doubt, that if I had ever attempted suicide, I would have succeeded.

I first became entirely aware of the idea of suicide when I was around nine and a half years old. A second cousin of mine did succeed in committing suicide, and strangely enough, I was not scared by the thought, but was curious. This was much like the curiosity I had about drugs. Even at that young age I was suicidal without even knowing it, or even really knowing what suicide was. This suicidal feeling was not the result of depression or a desire to end my suffering (at that time my illness was not yet causing me to suffer very much), but an example of the bizarre thinking that schizophrenia causes.

Another thing that fascinated me was the story of Judas Iscariot's suicide in the Bible. I was intrigued with the idea that I could cause my own death. At this time I had only known two people who had died, one of my grandfathers, and my second cousin that committed suicide (Elvis doesn't count because I didn't know him personally). I was interested in death, specifically my death, and the idea that I had the power to cause my own death.

Shortly after the death of my second cousin, I watched the TV miniseries *Shogun*. Throughout this miniseries, I watched a number of samurai committed *seppuku* (*hara-kiri*). By this time the symptoms of my illness were beginning to bother me, and suicide was becoming more and more appealing. A couple of times I considered committing seppuku, once I even held a hunting knife to my abdomen, but I just couldn't force the knife into me.

Slowly over time I became increasingly depressed, and over and over again I would seriously contemplate suicide. Most of the time it was over an unhappy incident that the idea of suicide would enter my mind, such as an argument with my parents, or the break up of a relation with a girlfriend, but many times it was just the schizophrenic torture building up in my head.

The first half a dozen years of my relationship with my wife soothed my schizophrenic torture and decreased my desire for suicide. I was still inundated with the symptoms of my illness, but any suicidal episodes didn't last long. The responsibility of having a wife and kids, as well as having the concrete love of a wife and kids, removed the thoughts of suicide from my head. I thought that I had reached a point in my emotional healing where suicide was no longer a danger.

During this time, a cousin of mine committed suicide. At that time I believed that I simply had a few emotional problems, of which I was working through, and that my cousin was following me, only he didn't get a chance work through his problems.

> Little brother don't dream my dream,
> Stay away it's a bad scene.
> Little brother you're out of control,
> You're in danger of losing your soul.
> I lived my life as if no one would care,
> Not realising someone was there.
> I turned my back on all that was true,
> Not thinking you would follow me too.
> Little brother don't dream my dream,
> Stay away it's a bad scene.
> Little brother you're out of control,
> You're in danger of losing your soul.
> I loved you more then I realised,
> I wish I told you before you died.
> I woke up and began to run,

But you kept dreaming 'til the dream was done.
Little brother don't dream my dream,
Stay away it's a bad scene.
Little brother you're out of control,
You're in danger of losing your soul.

My cousin's suicide upset me a great deal. It was like a portion of my childhood was destroyed.

I remember warm bright summers,
Climbing mountains made of sand.
Brave the cold wind for a ride down hill.
How I wish I was there still.
I thought our fun would last forever,
I thought we'd always stay the same.
But we grew up and now the hands of time
Have stopped our fun and changed the rhyme.
I thought our fun would last forever.
I thought we'd always stay the same.
I never thought the life you lived would be in vain.
I never thought you'd cause me so much pain.
Camping out in the mountains,
Telling stories by the fire,
Playing hide-and-seek in our grandma's trees,
Flying kites in the cool autumn breeze.
You left this all as nothing,
As if my love for you was gone.
But as the cold wind blew by your graveside,
A special part of me died.
I thought our fun would last forever.
I thought we'd always stay the same.
I never thought the life you lived would be in vain.
I never thought you'd cause me so much pain.

I remember all the good things,
My love for you will never end.
I'll think of all the fun we had,
I'll think of you and I'll not be sad.

At the time of his suicide, I was not suffering from suicidal thoughts. I believed that I was addressing my emotional problems, and resolving them. I wished that I had been able to talk to my cousin before he committed suicide. I also wanted to talk to other people before they attempt suicide. I thought I could say to them that I knew what you're going through, and that there was hope.

I come here as a friend, to say this ain't the end.
I know what you're going through,
and this ain't the thing to do.
I've stood where you now stand, held the gun in my hand,
Want the freedom found in death, praying for my final breath.
But there's one thing you must know, before you decide to go,
This life we live's not ours. It's the same as the wild flowers.
Our Father up above, He can fill you with his love,
Right your every wrong, and fill your soul with song.
There's a land of endless sorrows,
But you don't have to stay there.
He'll heal all your tomorrows,
And He'll guide you everywhere.
I've said what I had to say. How I wish you would stay.
Put the lock back on the gun, from your path now you must run.
Let the Father heal your pain. He'll wipe away all stain.
Clean you with His Holy Son, the battle has been won.
There's a land of endless sorrows,
But you don't have to stay there.
He'll heal all your tomorrows,
And He'll guide you everywhere.

Since I wrote this, my uncle, the father of my cousin that committed suicide, also committed suicide. I am so sorry that I couldn't do anything to prevent this. I want you, the reader, to know that I know what it's like, and that you can find hope if you look hard enough for it. I pray that there are no more suicides in my family.

Well, my suicidal thoughts were not the result of emotional problems, but the symptoms of my mental illness. As time went on, my schizophrenic and depressive symptom began to come back stronger than ever. The first half a dozen years I spent with my wife were the happiest years of my life. The love we shared with each other and with our children over powered my mental illness, but as time went on, my mental illness began to over power this love. I could understand my suicidal thought when I was younger because of my emotional problems and my loneliness, but how could I be suicidal when I had the love of my wife and children, and the healing of most of my emotional problems.

I decided that I needed a change, so I left my old job to start a new one. At first this change helped, but after a couple of months, the suicidal thoughts came back even stronger.

I began to be suicidal pretty much 24 hours a day. I went to a doctor who gave me some antidepressants. I was also looking up information about mental illness on the Internet. I decided that my symptoms matched schizophrenia, but I kept this self-diagnosis to myself.

I couldn't work any more. I had no concentration. I was paranoid. I was scared.

I confided in my mother-in-law, who told my mother, who, with my wife, took me to the hospital.

As we were driving to the hospital, it was all I could do to stop myself from opening the door of the car and jumping out. I was almost completely out of control.

My mother told the nurse at the emergency desk that I was very suicidal, which gave us very fast service. They admitted me, and took me to the lock down ward. This is the ward that has a locked door, no door knobs, bathrooms that can be locked to keep patients out but patients couldn't lock themselves in, and cloths hooks that can only support a couple pounds of weight so no one can hang themselves on them.

I cannot remember when this started, but sometime before my hospitalisation my suicidal thinking was accompanied by homicidal thinking. There was no reason for these homicidal thoughts other than the bizarre thinking that accompanies schizophrenia.

Because of my suicidal and homicidal thinking, the safety of myself and others was my main concern. Some nights I would ask that my bathroom be locked so I couldn't drown myself in the toilet. Sometimes I would ask that my garbage can be taken away so I couldn't suffocate myself with the plastic bag.

One day I became very concerned that the nurses were unaware of how strong I was, and that I may hurt someone. I asked that two of them to come into my room so I could show them this. They called security, and lock the door between their desk area and the patients' area. When two large security guards came, they escorted my nurse into my room. I took off my pyjama top, and flexed my muscles to show them how strong I was (at that time I was in pretty good shape). My nurse asked me to make a verbal contract to not hurt anyone, which I made. Looking back now, I don't think I was actually in danger of hurting anyone, but I was just scared that I might.

Since my hospitalisations I have had varying degrees of suicidal and homicidal thoughts depending on how effective my medication is. As I'm writing these words I am not being bothered by either, but this can change. Before my last medication change, my suicidal thoughts were returning, which is why there was a change in my medication. I don't remember the last time I had homicidal thoughts, but I know that there is always the possibility that they may return.

Sometimes my suicidal thoughts have been caused by a desire to end my suffering, but mostly they have just been the result of the bizarre thinking caused by my mental illness. When I do think of suicide as a solution to my suffering, I don't so much actively think of committing suicide, but wishing that suicide was a rational option.

Now that I've gone through what I've gone though, I'm not concerned about my suicidal and homicidal thoughts. When I had these thoughts my main concern was always my safety and the safety of others. I've never followed through, nor have I even begun to follow through, with any plans to commit suicide or homicide. I'm sure I will never follow through with either.

Now that I know that these are symptoms of my illness, I can talk myself through suicidal and homicidal episodes. I can objectively look at my thoughts and say to my self that this is just my illness, and it will pass. This is something that gives me great consolation: it's not me, it's my illness.

Bricks

I can really relate to the Pick Floyd movie, *The Wall*; however, this movie does give a false impression about mental illness. This movie seems to imply that life's experiences, especially childhood ones, can build a brick wall around someone and create a mental illness. This is not true. Mental illness is not caused by life's experiences, but is a disease that one is born with. While life's experience may contribute a brick or two, the illness itself builds the wall.

Throughout this book I've alluded to the wall that has surrounded me, cutting me off from the rest of humanity. This wall has given me very, very profound loneliness, but at the same time, has allowed me to function in society with an untreated mental illness for quite a long time. I believe that it was because of my attempt to destroy this wall that I ended up in the hospital's mental ward. If I had been content to remain completely alone, I could have lived my entire life without medical help.

I didn't want to remain completely alone. I wanted to experience love, and so the wall had to come down, and with it, my ability to cope with my illness.

This wall prevented me from absorbing the love and attention of my parents, as it did the love and attention of everyone else. From the beginning of elementary school, and possibly before, and into junior high school, I didn't fit into society. I had no real friends. My terrible time in grade seven was the greatest exemplification of this friendlessness. It was not that I didn't want friends, but that I didn't know how to function normally in society, and thus, couldn't make any friends. In addition to this, I also had the paranoid suspicion that no one really liked me, and were acting against me.

Starting around grade five and throughout junior high I learned a very important thing, non-verbal communication. Part of the school curriculum examined the way people, specifically North American people, communicated non-verbally. This curriculum taught me all the things that normal people would learn naturally without knowing it, such as when to make eye contact, for how long to make eye contact, and shifting your weight to one side when you want to terminate a conversation. I learned how to communicate this way, and also how to read the way others were communicating to me. Although I learned how to do this, and have become quite good at it, it still seems artificial and forced to me.

My bad experience in grade seven forced me to learn how to fit in. In grades eight and nine I attempted to fit in, albeit a bad attempt that relied on a large façade. By the time I started high school, I began to truly fit in, and by the end of high school, I was somewhat popular, and had a large number of acquaintances. I use the word *acquaintances* and not *friends* because of all these people, I now only have close contact with two of them, one of which I married.

It was through the relationship with my wife that I began to dismantle the wall around me, brick by brick. I wanted to dismantle the wall, but subconsciously I knew that the wall kept me safe. I thought that the wall I was dismantling was one created by emotional problems, and not one caused by mental illness. Before we were married, I did begin to open up a little, and I did tell my wife some of the bizarre things I've done. Once we were married, I also began to open up to my mother-in-law.

By socialising with my wife's family and extended family, I learned how to socialise. I do remember one occasion were I was forced into a social situation that I was not ready to embrace. We had a rather big party for my daughter's first birthday, and I was to play the part of host. I didn't know how to play this part, nor did I want to. I hid in the bathroom, until my wife angrily told me to get out. She was mad because her father and uncle had to take over the role I was supposed to play. Once I did join the party, I played the part of guest; the role of host was too much for me at that time. I did eventually learn how to play the role of host, but again, it seems forced and artificial.

It was the suicide of my cousin that jolted me into the decision to completely dismantle my wall. I did not want time to slip away without connecting with the people I love.

> I loved you more then I realised,
> I wish I told you before you died.

It was not too difficult to connect with my wife and kids, and even my in-laws, but I had a lifetime of being disconnected with my parents and sister to overcome. The big hurtle was to actually say, "I love you," to all three of them. I successfully jumped this hurtle all three times, but that was just the beginning.

After making sure I could express my love to everyone close to me, I started to focus on some of the bizarre things I've done. The first thing I focused on was my sexual past. I sought help from some professionals as well as my mom and my mother-in-law.

Once I began to have some healing in this area I thought I was almost done dealing with all the emotional garbage of my past. I was almost done with my emotional garbage, but just beginning on my mental illness garbage. Working out one's emotional garbage is quite different than dealing with a mental illness.

Talking about it didn't seem to help, but seemed to make it worse. People have told me that they could start to see that something was wrong with me the summer before my first hospitalisation. One clue was that I got a little bit drunk at a wedding, something which was out of character for me. What I was dealing with at the time I could not talk about. No human language can fully express what was going through my head.

The wall was beginning to crumble, and I couldn't control it anymore.

The wall was destroyed the day I was admitted into the hospital. I talked freely about anything and everything. I'm sure I made some of my visitors quite uncomfortable with what I had to say, both about me and about them.

I'm not sure whether it's fortunate or unfortunate that I can't remember much about my hospitalisations or the time in-between them. Anyway, I can't say anymore about the wall coming down because I don't remember anymore.

Since my second, and hopefully my last, hospitalisation I have begun to rebuild my wall. This time I'm building a healthy wall. There are a number of things that I want others to know about me, but there are other things that I should only share with a few specially chosen people, such as my mental health nurse and my doctor. When my wall was completely down I had no discretion. I'd talk about anything to anyone. Such an action is not socially acceptable.

Now that I know that I have a mental illness, and what its symptoms are, I can let the appropriate people know what symptoms are affecting me, but I have enough of a wall to limit this to the appropriate people. However, I must be careful not to put too many bricks in this wall.

Barbwire

When Jesus Christ was being tortured before His crucifixion, a crown of thorns was placed on His head; throughout my schizophrenic torture I have worn a similarly symbolic crown made of barbwire. This crown had caused be a great deal of pain; as well, due to being made of metal, it short-circuits the signals in my brain, causing unusual and bizarre thinking and behaviour. The only consolation I have is that I can be united with Jesus in my suffering by wearing a crown similar to His.

I have lightly touched upon this topic in the other chapters of this book, but now I will go into a little more detail. While I can describe the bizarre things I've done, I cannot give a reason for doing these things, nor can I adequately describe the bizarre thoughts and feeling that I've had. Much of these thoughts and feelings are beyond human language. Nonetheless, I will attempt to describe them.

My inability to function in society is one of the biggest short-circuits in my brain. The way people naturally communicate with each other is often artificial and forced for me. This is coupled with profound loneliness and the feeling that no one really wants to be with me. Many times I have to objectively say to myself that people really do want to be with me, even though it doesn't seem like it to me. Now that I know that this is a symptom of my mental illness, I can work through it, but it still makes me feel lonely.

In addition to this, sometimes the tone in people's voices can shut me down. This tone is somewhat of a lecturing tone, and it causes me to stop sending and receiving communication. Often this was the tone teachers used with me, and really, they could have just as well been talking to a brick wall. There was one occasion at work where a co-worker was supposed to spend a few days teaching me how use a particular software development kit (a computer thingy), but because of his tone of voice, I could have gotten just as much out of it as if I didn't come in for work on those days. Actually, this tone doesn't have to be directed at me. I will shut down even when someone else is being talked to in this tone.

I've seen a lecture on video by a person with schizophrenia who talked about the same thing. He says that he carries some cards with him that basically say, "Because of my mental illness, I cannot continue this conversation with the tone of voice you are using." When a person starts talking to him in this particular tone, he gives them one of these cards. He gives out the cards because he can't even tell the person what this tone of voice is doing to him.

Obviously my homicidal and suicidal thoughts are a result of the barbwire's short-circuiting. Fortunately I've never attempted to follow through with these thoughts. They used to scare me, but now I can simply say to myself that it's part of my illness, and it will eventually pass.

I've already talked about how, at times, it seem that different objects are controlling me. This is why I burnt different objects, such as my books by J. R. R. Tolkien, and many of my records, to free me from their control. As well, I sometimes feel that other people are controlling me. Again, I'm not talking about normal control, but the type of control as if they are manipulating the thoughts in my head.

One such controlling experience that has been very prevalent in my life has been the idea that my life is an experiment. Someone, or possibly everyone other than me, is conducting an experiment on me to see how I will react to everything around me. I'm not sure whether other people are also being experimented on, or whether everyone is just acting as controlled variables in the experiment. This is one thing that can also cause me to think of suicide. If I kill myself, I'd stop the experiment.

I actually talked to one of the other patients about this during my first hospitalisation. I really like this one patient, although he never said much that made any sense. It seemed to me that he spoke in metaphors, although I may have been the only one that recognised this. Anyway, I thought I could trust him. While we were alone in the TV area, which was also the smoking area and was glassed off from the main area on the ward were nobody could here us talk, I asked him if he thought we were in an experiment. I took a bit of time and explained exactly what I meant. He didn't say much at the time, but the next day he basically told me that what we were talking about the day before was entirely crazy. This was the most coherent thing he ever said to me, and so I thought I was safe and was not part of a big experiment.

I also have the opposite experience to that of thinking my life is an experiment, where I think everything is not real. It seems kind of like a dream. This type of feeling can give me somewhat of a high, because it gives me the feeling that I can manipulate things with my mind. This type of feeling can make me feel good because it gives me some power, but I have to be careful and forcefully tell myself that this is all in my head.

Another experience that is similar to thinking everything is not really real, is thinking I'm not really where I seem to be. It's as if I'm living in a hallucination. My senses tell me I'm in one place, while in reality I'm somewhere else. The most common example of this that has been occurring to me since I was quite young is that I think I'm in church, but really I'm in my mom's garden. I sit, stand, and sing in church, but in reality I'm sitting, standing, and singing in my mom's garden, which isn't too bad unless other people are watching me do this. Again, I can talk myself through this. I know I'm really in church, and this feeling will pass.

These last three experiences, the experiment, things aren't real, and I'm not really where I am, all involve paranoia to some degree. I've also had intense paranoia on its own, especially just before my first hospitalisation. I would actually be constantly looking over my shoulders to see if anyone was watching me. I became very uncomfortable with my cubical at work because I had my back to a window. I still get this a fair bit. Often I'm overly cautious that nobody can see what my locker combination is at the gym; I'll check every room in the house to make sure I'm really alone; and sometimes I feel that the people around me can see the thoughts that are going through my mind, which is very unnerving.

Some people will actually have auditory and visual hallucinations with schizophrenia; fortunately, I've had neither of these. What I have had is voices in my head. These voices are only in my head, they are not auditory. They also speak another language that I cannot understand, although I understand the feelings they convey. When I was very young, these voices would come, but they would be somewhat comforting. As I grew up these voices slowly changed from being comforting to being disturbing and tormenting. Before my first hospitalisation, these voices were becoming unbearable.

Another thing that has been at times very unbearable is severely intense anxiety. Anytime I had to do anything out of the ordinary, I would become very anxious. That is, more than normal. An example of this was when some friends of mine were putting on a musical performance during lunch hour in high school. I was only in the audience and not doing anything special; however, I was so anxious that I was actually shaking. It was all I could do to conceal my shaking.

Related to anxiety is something my mental health nurse and I call *the sidewalk experience*. I would describe it as the physically manifestation of anxiety. This feeling stems from a nightmare I would have when I was around five until the middle of elementary school. In this dream, I'm walking fast down a sidewalk. I have to hurry because I have to save the world. The world and everything in it is about to expand until it explodes, unless I stop it. As I'm walking, the sidewalk begins to expand. I pass by a policeman who holds out a flower to me, but the flower begins to expand. I never reach the end of the sidewalk, and things just keep expanding and get more and more intense. This dream would create a very powerful bout of anxiety. Now that I'm older, I don't have this dream, but I do get the same feeling that this dream invoked while I'm awake. It's difficult to adequately describe this feeling in words. It's such an intense feeling that suicide almost seems reasonable to stop it.

Delusional thinking is also associated with schizophrenia, and I've had a great deal of this. At times, it has been very strong, but most of the time it has been very subtle. I would some how think that I had priority over everyone else. I would hoard things, and even steal things, but all along I always thought I was justified.

I would also lie. I believed that by changing a story or a fact it would become truth. Many times it was obvious that I was lying, which only made me look foolish and dishonest.

During my first hospitalisation I became very delusional. I don't remember much of it, but I do know that I believed God was talking to me. People have told me that I believed that I didn't have to eat anymore; I believed that God would sustain me without earthly food. I also believed that I would die if I didn't receive communion every day. Fortunately I had a priest friend that would bring me communion on Saturdays when the regular people that distributed communion in the hospitable didn't come.

Another delusional thought is that I can reach some sort of mystical unity with the world by attempting to become one with nature. Since I grew up on a farm I would often go for walks in the woods. When this delusional thought would come to me, I would take off all of my clothes, my earrings, my glasses, and anything else that is unnatural. I would attempt to be completely physically and mentally one with nature. I would not do this for very long since I can't see more than a foot in front of my face without my glasses.

Often this thought of mystically becoming united with the world was accompanied with the idea that some power was leading me as I walked. I would wander without having a destination other than the unknown destination that the power leading me had in store. This became more prevalent once I started college and working in the city. I would wander aimlessly through the streets of the city not knowing where my destination was. When I wandered through the streets of the city, I would not take off my cloths, although a few times I would take of my watch, wedding ring, necklace, earrings, and anything else nonessential.

While I wandered aimlessly through the streets of the city, I would be off in my own little world, withdrawn from society. Most of the time during these episodes I was unable to study or work, as well as being unable to deal with social contact.

From elementary school to high school, I would do the same thing, only instead of aimlessly walking through the town streets I would stay home from school, and withdraw into my bedroom. I was not physically sick, but was mentally sick, and I just couldn't deal with society, so I stayed home from school to be by myself in my bedroom.

Because I was staying home from school a lot, I would be constantly going to different doctors. Most of the time they couldn't find anything wrong with me since the trouble was not physical but mental (It should be noted that mental illnesses are physical illnesses, but they are not yet detectable like other physical illnesses). Occasionally I would have some physical symptoms, but I think most of the time these physical symptoms were caused by my mental illness.

Staying home from school also gave me a great deal of problems in school. Most of my junior high school teachers didn't know how to grade me because I missed most of the assignments and tests. My mom would bring work home for me, but most of the time I didn't do it. The pressure to be social and to study was too much for me to handle.

One day in grade nine, I was called to the office to meet with the principal, and if I remember correctly, one of the vice-principals, as well as someone from the school board. They knew something was wrong and they wanted to help me. I completely shut down, and gave them no information. I couldn't tell them anything. I began to cry, and they asked me why I was crying, but I couldn't tell them. I really didn't know myself. They eventually gave up, and told me to clean myself up in the bathroom and go back to class.

Staying home all the time and not doing my homework gave me a very negative self-image. I believed I was lazy and worthless. Even when I forced myself to work hard in college and at work, I would have bouts where I couldn't work, which I interpreted as laziness. It was a big relief for me when I realised that I was not lazy, but was mentally ill, and that I did the best I could to deal with this illness, especially in college where I received an honours diploma.

One of the most bizarre things I've done is self-mutilation. I have around a half dozen scars on my chest from cutting myself on different occasions with razor blades. One of these scars is two inches long and is quite visible. As well, I used to take sewing needles and push them deep into my skin. I can't explain why I did these things; I can only attribute this bizarre behaviour to my illness.

All of this bizarre thinking and the other thing I've mentioned in this book have caused me a great deal of pain and suffering. To escape from my painful reality, I have a very vivid and extensive fantasy life. As I said earlier, I would miss a lot of school, and I would spend most of this free time laying on my bed imagining a better life for myself. I would imagine the most minuscule details, and at times even have the delusional belief that these fantasies could come true.

In recent years, I have tried to minimise this fantasy life and spend my time in more productive ways, such as writing this book. But force of habit and the pain of my illness do cause me to spend at least some of my time fantasizing a better life for myself.

My crown of barbwire is painful, but I lift up my pain to God, and I pray that myself and others will benefit from this pain.

Appendix: Feelings Scale

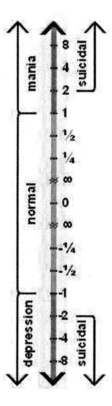

This is a scale to rate where your feelings are. There is no such thing as a good feeling or a bad feeling; all feelings are neutral. Feelings are neither positive nor negative, but abstract. For this scale, I use the terms positive and negative not for good and bad, but for their quantitative characteristics. It is good to know what your feelings are, especially if you are suffering from a mental illness.

I came up with this *Feeling Scale* during my first hospitalisation. While in the hospital the staff would ask me to rate my feelings on a scale from zero to ten. This made no sense to me. Did zero mean a normal low or the most clinically depressed low possible? If zero was a normal low, how do you rate a clinically depressed low? If zero was the lowest clinically depressed low, what was a normal low? I would guess around four, as you can get quite low with clinical depression. The same could also be said for the highs and mania. The only number I was sure of was five. It is right in the middle but that was not how I felt most of the time.

I decided zero must be the middle of the scale, as it signifies true nothing, neither positive nor negative. With zero in the middle, this allows positive and negative numbers to describe my feelings. This leaves us with the question of where this scale ends. To keep it short, it doesn't. Both the positive and negative ends of the scale continue into infinity. This makes complete sense when you consider that everyone is different and dips higher or lower than others towards infinite depression and mania.

Now where do we draw the line between normal feelings and exaggerated or mentally ill feelings? 'One' is the number that means total or complete, so positive one and negative one is where a persons feelings leaves the normal healthy range and enters the dangerous region.

At some point on the scale, suicide becomes a very real danger. It is possible to be depressed or manic beyond the point of normal and not be suicidal, so the first step past positive or negative one is marked as being suicidal. The point of having suicidal thoughts can be anywhere on the scale; however, at positive or negative two there is the danger of acting on these thoughts.

When people are past positive one and negative one, things seem to get out of control very fast. This is why the scale is exponential. This also shows how close suicide can be to a total but normal high or low. The distance between positive and negative one and zero is infinitely greater than the distance between positive and negative one and the suicidal positive and negative two. This should show how fast a depressed person can become a danger to him or herself.

The following formulas describe the different ranges of feelings, which can also be very useful in describing a person's feelings. These formulas describe a normal range of feelings, an abnormal range of feelings, or such a rapid change of feelings that you cannot put a number on it. For these formulas, the variable f represents the numerical value of a person's feelings.

$-1 \leq f \leq +1$

This is the normal and healthy range of feelings. You can still have a problem in this range if your feelings are not changing slowly and smoothly. This is not to say that you cannot have a sudden change of feelings, but you should not rapidly change between positive and negative feelings more than a couple times in quick succession.

$-1 > f > +1$

This is the abnormal or unhealthy range of feelings. When a person is only in this range, he skips over the normal range ($-1 \leq f \leq +1$) when going from negative to positive or positive to negative. This problem can be compounded by rapid changes between positive and negative.

$0 \geq f \geq 0$ or $-\infty < f < +\infty$

This is still an abnormal range of feelings; however, the normal range of feelings can still be reached. Again, this problem can be compounded by rapid changes between positive and negative.

For me this is a more accurate way of describing my feelings than a scale of zero to ten. The scale of zero to ten may still be an easier way for many people to describe their feelings; however, my scale is the only logical way for me to describe my feelings.

Printed in the United States
23602LVS00001B/793-840